NATURAL SOLUTIONS FOR YOUR CHILD AND FAMILY

Natural Solutions for Your Child and Family

A Pediatrician's Path to Wellness

Ruth M. Rodriguez, DO

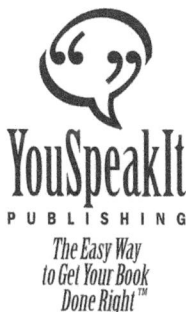

YouSpeakIt
PUBLISHING
*The Easy Way
to Get Your Book
Done Right*™

ISBN: 978-1-945446-72-6

This book is dedicated to all children, former and future patients, and clients I have been blessed and honored to serve. You have all been my inspiration, my fire to learn more about the many ways to support and help you with all-natural solutions.

Contents

CHAPTER FIVE

Acknowledgments

I'd like to acknowledge all parents and caretakers of children who are looking for natural solutions as alternatives for their health and wellness. I appreciate you all so very much.

I want to acknowledge the many mentors and leaders before me as well as other like-minded, health-conscious individuals who are currently helping others with plant-based nutrition, medicines, products, mindsets, and affirmations to improve children's health and protect our planet.

I also want to acknowledge Babypie Publishing and their YouSpeakIt program for making my dream of a published book a reality; the process was joyful and everyone involved helped to make it an easy one.

I'd like to say a great big thank you to my three endorsers of this book: AmondaRose Igoe, Anthony Profeta, and Scott Donat. I so appreciated your support and guidance to get this book out to the readers.

I would also like to thank my mentor, Gina Devee of Divine Living Academy, whose faith-based guidance has inspired me both personally and professionally.

Last but not least, I'd like to thank my mother and father, my two daughters, and my new husband; their unconditional love and emotional support always provide the solid foundation

I need in my life and have helped me get this project off the ground.

I am eternally grateful for all of you, the reader, because you have given me more than you could ever imagine!

Introduction

This book relates my personal and professional struggles as a pediatrician, mom, and marathon runner. While I understood the connection between emotional traumas in my personal life and getting sick frequently, even with my knowledge and experience as a Western medicine physician, I was unable to effectively heal myself. Additionally, I was concerned about the negative side effects of certain medications. I knew that many of them contain toxic ingredients that could harm me.

At the same time, I became increasingly aware of the damage we cause to our planet by using artificial, manufactured, and toxic products, as well as pesticides used in conventionally grown foods. I also became aware of the damage caused by the additives used in processed foods and other products and how they were affecting my patients' health. Everything we put on, and in, our bodies affects our health and our planet.

When I was a child, my grandmother used all-natural remedies every time I got sick. But on the other end of the spectrum, my father took me to the pharmacist with a prescription for antibiotics every time I had a common childhood illness. I saw the dichotomy.

The Hippocratic Oath requires physicians to do no harm to our patients. So, I made it my life's passion and mission to lead parents in helping them heal their children with all-natural, nontoxic remedies.

I continue to learn something new every day in my search for better health, and I feel blessed to have acquired this knowledge. I want to share it with others to improve our children's health and help parents on this journey. Together we can minimize and move toward completely alleviating the damage we inflict on our planet. It's also a way to give back to Divinity for blessing us with the opportunity to live and share with each other.

If you decide to work with me and you are a parent, you will get the best of my knowledge. I will leave no stone unturned to help find easy and healthy solutions for your child. These may include simple lifestyle changes and creating a customized wellness plan that works best for your child and your family.

I will look for the root cause of your child's problem. I will incorporate emotional affirmations into your child's healing program as well.

Whether or not you choose to work with me, I believe you will gain invaluable knowledge from this book about the connection of emotions and diseases, natural remedies, toxic ingredients and their negative side effects that you may not be aware of, and comprehensive information about our connection to Divinity and our responsibility to our planet.

CHAPTER ONE

My Story and Ideas

Ask, and it will be given you. Seek, and you will find.
Knock, and it will be opened for you.
Matthew 7:7, WEB

BACKGROUND: AWARENESS

I was born in Santa Clara, Cuba. My journey to the United States took place with my parents and my sister when I was seven years old. At the time, it was known as one of the hundreds of thousands of Freedom Flights. During the 1960s, hundreds of thousands of Cubans came to the United States. We arrived with resident status, and after five years, we became American citizens.

My drive for excellence, my will for learning, and my goal orientation stem from this experience.

It truly was a defection from our country for a much better life, and it shaped the person I am today. As a child, I remember feeling fear of the unknown future, and the loss of what I had known—my life in Cuba. But, I was a child, so I had a lot of acceptance; I had no judgment of the situation, and I was happy, hopeful, and positively anticipating the new life I was about to experience.

That was the foundation from which I built my life. I tried to see every situation without judgment, and remain optimistic, in spite of the dramatic experience of being plucked from the country of my birth and moved to a new country without knowing the language and without the support of my friends, the rest of my family, and other loved ones. Once we received our notice in the mail, we had four days to prepare to leave the country and make our flight to the United States. I have never gone back to Cuba since then because of Cuba's policies against those who left before 1971 and other humanitarian reasons.

It was a miracle to come to this country with resident status—which, I believe, has never, ever happened in the history of United States with any other country and hasn't happened since. It was a living miracle for me to be part of that and for which I am grateful to the U.S.A. and Divinity.

How the Move Shaped My Life

That experience was stressful for all members of my family, including me, because it was a complete change from what we had previously known; we had moved to a life of unknowns. But we all had accepting views, and we were optimistic, especially because we knew we would be American citizens in five years. And at the five-year mark, all four of us proudly became citizens.

Because we had resident status, my father was able to work. He was effective at that and quickly found a full-time construction job and set up his own after-hours office-cleaning business. We knew he would provide for us.

My mother also learned the language and went back to school to get her teaching license in the U.S.A. She was an elementary school ESOL (English for Speakers of Other Languages) teacher and taught my sister and me how to read and write in Spanish after hours at home.

I had a very strict upbringing. Because of that, and because my parents had a fear of strangers, I grew up with a lot of cultural ideas, many of which were simply untrue. For example, I was warned that strangers might give me the evil eye. I was warned not to swim after meals, which is a common myth in many cultures. But, we loved going to the beach on Sundays, and we were not supposed to swim for two hours after we ate. I had to be chaperoned while on dates in high school and college.

There were many cultural ideas like not swimming after meals; for example, being careful not to get exposed to cold air after showers to avoid getting a cold, and not breathing or talking in cold wind while walking outside since that may cause you to catch a cold. I was also verbally and physically disciplined. It was a worrisome and fearful upbringing, but I understand that it was the cultural norm at the time.

When I was around ten years old, I had a near-drowning experience. I remember three times going underwater while my father sensed I was missing and then saw me moving farther and farther away in the ocean. All of a sudden, my dad swam up to me and brought me to shore. The loss of control in that incident was a transformational experience for me. Afterward, I recall being brought back to safety and the feeling of life and health again. I think that helped me become much more aware of my body and my health, as well as our vulnerability and our connection to Spirit.

I remember asking God to save me. I remember seeing the shoreline getting farther and farther away, panicking, and giving up as well.

The experience was stressful but I learned from it. I also learned valuable lessons from other experiences I had while growing up in Miami, and I learned from the experiences of other family members as well—how they assimilated and adapted in their migration journey.

Being with my grandmother was also transformational for me. My grandmother was a very spiritual person who showed me what unconditional love is. She had a lot of cultural ideas of spirituality, like prayer to the Sacred Heart of Jesus. She recited a special chant every time she lost an item—more of a chanting dance for lost things. I grew up with this spirituality instilled in me.

My grandmother was also the basis for my ideas of natural remedies. She always tried teas and herbs when someone in the family got sick.

Through my father, I learned about the importance of health. The near-drowning experience and the loss of control I felt when that happened helped me realize I could take control of my health, but our *existence* is not in our control. There's a living spirit guiding and supporting us. My father was very germ-phobic, and he was always reading about natural remedies and how to keep yourself healthy.

I had a loving relationship with my father, more like a friendship between equals than a father-daughter relationship. He was the one who nurtured me growing up. He was very comical, so we shared a lot of laughter together.

My mother was spiritual, faith-based, disciplined, and clean. I learned from my sister to be studious and to strive for educational excellence, to be goal-oriented and result-driven.

Upbringing Leads to Desire to Help Children

Through my upbringing and the lessons I learned from my other family members, I developed my own approach to life. My desire to become a pediatrician stemmed initially from wanting to help other children have this approach to life: a combination of spirituality and faith, mindset and hope, and health.

In the area of health, I achieved control through physical exercise and positive affirmations. Emotions play a vital part in our health, and in my role as pediatrician, I want to help other people with that mindset.

As a mother of two, another reason for becoming a pediatrician was to help other mothers learn about the three basic foundations that rule my life:

- Spirituality
- Mindset
- Health and Body

I pray every day, and I also ask God a lot of questions. Each day, I read new information from many sources. I always do my best to stay positive. I have a regular routine of physical activity. I attend to my emotional health with positive affirmations. These practices keep me goal- and results-oriented, so I always have something to look forward to.

My message is one of guiding people to stay positive, to keep moving forward, and to stay goal- and results-oriented.

> *I can do all things through Christ who strengthens me.*
> Philippians 4:13, NIV

PEDIATRIC TRAINING AND EXPERIENCE: DISCOVERY

The reason I want to share about my training and experience as a pediatrician is because it opened my mind to all the different ways we can help our children with their health.

Traditional Western Medicine

I was trained in traditional Western medicine, and I learned a lot of traditional ways of treating diseases based on symptoms, diagnoses, prescriptions, and OTC medications; but because of my background and upbringing with natural remedies, I became aware that my experience in a traditional setting was more and more out of alignment.

I chose Western medicine because of my dad; he was the one who influenced me to choose my career. He always wanted to be a physician himself, but he didn't have the opportunity. He read about natural remedies, and, as mentioned, was germ-phobic and health-oriented. He instilled in me the desire to reach for the stars.

When he dropped me off at medical school, he looked me in the eye on my first day and said, "Pretend you are in jail, Ruth, for the next four years."

"What do you mean?" I asked.

"This is the only way you are going to get through this. It is pure sacrifice, dedication, and goal orientation for the next four years. Don't focus on anything else but getting through medical school."

In my mind at the time, it was the ultimate success to complete my education in traditional Western medicine. I had arrived as a little girl in what my family and I consider to be the greatest country of all and was on a journey to become a respected medical doctor.

Awareness of Traditional Medicine

I have been a pediatrician for twenty-four years, a solo pediatrician in private practice for fifteen of those years. Through these years in the office, I have had a lot of one-on-one doctor-patient relationships with families. I became increasingly aware that the medications I was prescribing to them, and sometimes even over-the-counter (OTC) medications, were giving my patients negative side effects from toxic ingredients.

This led me to go back to my upbringing with natural remedies and to do research. Through my research, I discovered other effective options I could use to help patients while relieving their worry about negative side effects from the toxins.

The Hippocratic Oath came to mind: *Do no harm.*

Seeing patients with negative side effects due to toxic ingredients in the medications I was prescribing brought that home, and it bothered me that I was not being true to my oath to do no harm.

Natural Medicine

I am an osteopath, a Doctor of Osteopathy, not an MD. They also teach us osteopathic manipulations in medical school. We learn how the musculoskeletal system is involved in disease processes and how diseases affect the musculoskeletal system. Because of learning about osteopathic manipulation, I am open to alternative medicine modalities such as acupuncture, chiropractic treatment, and natural remedies. I was not directly taught any natural remedies, but I was always open to this because of my grandmother's influence.

As mentioned, I was seeing the negative side effects from toxic ingredients in the patients I was treating. I also went through my own health crisis when I was diagnosed with a serious sinus infection called *pansinusitis,* which is an infection of all eight sinuses. I was hospitalized for five days.

After I was released from the hospital, I was on multiple medications, and I had side effects from each one. When I looked up each medication I was prescribed, I read the potential side effects, and I experienced one or more from each.

That set me on the path of researching alternatives and discovering natural remedies. I had read as much as I could, watched videos, gone to classes offered in the area, professional classes offered outside the area—basically consumed any information I could find that advised the use of natural or alternative remedies.

I attended homeopathy conferences, functional medicine conferences, and learned about essential oils. I went on a quest. For more than two years, I have actively been on this quest of discovering more natural remedies, including acupuncture, acupressure, and Reiki healing. I am still constantly researching and learning more every day. I am also familiar with positive affirmations. I have been able to use all these at various times to improve my own health, my family's health, and my patients' health.

NATURAL MEDICINE: SHIFT

I want to share with you the many different alternative medicines you can use to heal yourself and to heal your children. With Western medicine, there is only one main set of principles for doing things, which is treating symptoms, often with prescribed drugs.

Natural medicine, on the other hand, may include:

- Homeopathy
- Essential oils
- Herbal medicine
- Chinese medicine
- Acupuncture

- Chiropractic
- Reiki
- Reflexology
- Meditation
- Prayer
- Affirmations
- Mantras

Discovering natural medicine was like discovering a fountain of wisdom because it opened all possibilities and a variety of paths to follow for optimum health. It also allowed me to treat myself and my patients effectively without the worry of negative side effects or toxic ingredients, and most importantly, it allowed me to do no harm to our bodies and our planet.

Transition and Challenge

The challenge of natural medicine for me personally has been learning how to transition from Western medicine to natural remedies and how to easily incorporate alternatives within my current profession.

Three years ago, I closed down my office, and I became employed by a large hospital corporation that contracts with two local hospitals. Since that time, I have worked as a pediatric hospitalist. This position involves taking care of children when they are in the hospital overnight.

Over the past year, I have been traveling as a pediatric hospitalist, substituting for other doctors in clinics, nurseries, and pediatric floors in many hospitals all around the U.S.A. My challenge is to help families using natural remedies in a hospital setting where there are set rules and regulations because these hospitals are based on traditional Western medicine principles. As a hospital employee, it has been a challenge to share my knowledge of natural therapies with families whose children are under my charge, unless the family asks me directly to recommend natural remedies.

Essentially, families must approach me and ask what I would do if my own child were sick, or what I would do outside of the traditional Western medicine approach.

Applying New Methods

It soon became my goal to share the enormous value that can be gained by finding and applying natural medicine alternatives. And that's why I'm sharing what I have learned about natural medicine with you through this book.

Results

The first thing I noticed were the results I, myself, experienced using natural remedies. All the negative side effects I had been experiencing from prescribed medications were resolved, including the worry about the side effects. Additionally, I was soon relieved of the worry over toxic ingredients in manufactured medication, because natural remedies prescribed by a licensed, trained practitioner are much less likely to cause any damaging side effects.

The results have been excellent overall. In most cases, patients show marked improvement; and in all cases, using natural remedies has been worry-free. I have witnessed quick and effective physical and mental improvements in my patients' health. The results have been truly impressive.

Parents are not in a trial-and-error situation when working with me, or with anyone familiar with these natural alternative remedies and modalities I mentioned, as that simply isn't necessary with natural remedies. The remedy typically works the first or second time. That is quite unlike Western medicine and prescribed medications where trial and error is the norm.

Additionally, time is not wasted. Parents generally do not have to miss work, and children do not need to be away from school. With the shift to natural medicine, those absences are significantly diminished—if not eliminated entirely. With natural medicine, parents don't have to take time off from work to stay home with their child, and the child does not have to miss school because they get well so much more quickly.

Another benefit of shifting from Western medicine to natural medicine is saving money. Natural remedies are usually very economical compared to traditional Western medicine remedies.

CHAPTER TWO

Mindset and Emotions

Gracious words are like a honeycomb,
sweetness to the soul and health to the body.
Proverbs 16:24, ESV

MY JOURNEY

As I have already mentioned, I grew up in a household where my grandmother was the head of the house, and she was especially knowledgeable about nutrition and natural remedies including herbs, essential oils, and teas. Any time someone in the family was sick or had some sort of ailment, the solution would be found in a natural remedy.

During my training as a physician, my grandmother's alternative methods stayed with me in the background. Even today, I always search for the least invasive way of treating patients, especially young children.

In my own practice, I recommended a variety of natural remedies, and I made use of several myself for my own health. These natural remedies include Vitamin C, saline nose washes, and gargling with salt water. These natural ways to improve my patients' health, as well as the health of my family, are due to my grandmother's influence.

How My Training and Experience Made Me Aware

My residency and hospital training as a pediatrician were Western-medicine based. During my experience in the office and hospital, I became increasingly aware of the negative side effects that patients were experiencing. Additionally, I began to understand and feel the repercussions of the toxic ingredients in the medications I was taking myself.

Making the Connection

I got sick. In my forties, I started getting increasingly unhappy with my personal home life and with my marriage. I felt emotionally disconnected from my husband. As I became increasingly sad and unhappy with my personal life, I noticed that every time a sick child would come into the office, my chance of catching that illness was growing exponentially.

When I had a bout of anxiety, a bout of crying over my marriage situation, or an argument with my husband, I would inevitably come into the office sad. Then, when I was exposed to a sick child in the office, I had a conscious feeling that I was going to get sick because I was so sad. It was a gut-wrenching feeling.

Sure enough, I would be sick a couple days later. The year prior to my divorce, I was sick five or six times. Once I became aware that this frequency in illness was caused by my emotions bringing down my immune system, I remembered the natural remedies that my grandmother recommended.

Sometimes I would combine the natural remedies with my traditional Western medicine training, and I would put myself on a course of antibiotics for five to ten days.

On one particular occasion, I put myself on antibiotics for much longer than would have been medically recommended, but it was the only thing I could see that would help me. Every ten days, I would give myself a different family of antibiotics. In medical school, they teach us that some antibiotics belong to the penicillin family or the cephalosporin family, so I would try a different type of antibiotic. I had a bad sinus infection, but it grew worse.

I hadn't yet made the connection between what was going on in my personal life and the lack of resolution for my sinus infection. My increasing frustration around not knowing the solution for my unhappy marriage was paralleled by the frustration of not being able to find a solution for my sinus infection.

Because of my strong work ethic derived from being born in another country, coming to the United States, and starting over from scratch, I continued to push myself to the limit with a move-ahead, never-ever-quit mentality.

I remember I continued to work and I also signed up for a half-marathon. I had been ill for at least two months, and I had a half-marathon coming up, which I didn't train properly for. But I went ahead and completed it.

The week after I returned, I went right back to work, and sure enough, I found myself on the couch one day, completely unable to stand up to drive myself to the office. I had met my own requirement for hospitalization. I had been up all night coughing.

I had been giving myself nebulizer treatments with Western medicine; I had exhausted all my knowledge of natural remedies; I was completely emotionally disconnected from my husband. I was in a very sad state with a low immune system as well. I was in the hospital for five days.

The week after my stay in the hospital, I went right back to working full-time. I noticed that I was experiencing side effects from the multiple medications I had taken during my hospital stay, a variety of antibiotics and steroids. I had side effects that I knew could be secondary to the medication, but I went a step further and looked them up.

Sure enough, each medication coincided with the side effect I was experiencing. They were scary to me. Once, while taking a nap, I dreamed of eating a metal can; when I woke up, I had a metallic taste in my mouth. That taste is a known side effect of the antibiotic I was taking.

While taking a different antibiotic, I felt joint pain while at rest, specifically in my Achilles tendon area. The antibiotic I was taking then is associated with tears to the Achilles tendon; people may experience severe pain in that area.

All the side effects made me wonder what I was doing to my body by consuming all these chemicals that were not natural. So, I decided to return to my grandmother's idea to let nature help; after all, fruits and vegetables—everything found in nature—were placed there by God and the Universe to help us.

Because I felt I had closed all the other doors I had been trying to go through with Western medicine, I went back to my grandmother's original idea. I started searching for natural remedies.

During this time, I would often go home during my lunch break so I could lie down in the hopes of regaining enough strength to make it through my afternoon. One day, I woke up from my nap and remembered I was an osteopath; it was like a flashlight lit up in my mind.

In osteopathic medical school, we were taught that bones and muscles in the body can be manipulated to help with diseases. My first thought was to get my sinuses and chest manipulated because I had a sinus infection and severe bronchitis. I began my search for other practitioners that did osteopathic manipulation.

I found a chiropractor who specialized in craniosacral manipulations. He recommended a natural nose wash that physically thins mucus, so I started that practice with a solution called *Alkalol,* an all-natural mucus solvent that has been around for over forty years.

Alkalol is mixed with saline, half and half. While holding my breath, I washed my nose with this half and half solution. This is how I slowly got over my sinus infection. I also stopped all prescription medications, antibiotics, and steroids, and had osteopathic and chiropractic manipulations in addition to the natural nose washes. I was better in no time. I quickly recuperated.

Since then, I have been conscious of what I put into my body and the products that I use. I am wary of something that is not natural-based because the body may or may not respond to it appropriately. Everything that is non-natural and man-made is going to have a potential side effect from the toxic ingredients. Natural remedies and therapies have much fewer negative side effects or toxic ingredients and are much less likely to cause harm.

The Law of Attraction and Mindset

I have always done a lot of reading and researching and have found a lot of helpful information over the years. During an Internet search, I discovered the prayer of Jabez. Because I was unhappy in my marriage, I also started praying this prayer.

A priest dedicated his entire life to teaching people about the power of this prayer. It's a one-paragraph section in the Bible:

> *Jabez cried out to the God of Israel, "Oh, that you would bless me and enlarge my territory! Let your hand be with me, and keep me from harm so that I will be free from pain." And God granted his request.*
>
> 1 Chronicles 4:10, NIV

The first part of the prayer is Jabez asking to be blessed; the second is praying for God to increase his territory, meaning that God is going to help you with whatever you wish or desire to create in your life. The third part of the prayer is not to have any harm come to you and, as I interpret it, for you not to cause anyone else harm.

That resonated with me as a server of health and clashed with my upbringing in the fatalistic idea that life happens to you, instead of life being created by you. This prayer was a nice way for me to transition into changing my mindset and positively taking more control of my own life. I prayed this prayer daily for an entire year, during all of 2009.

At the end of 2009, a girlfriend who is a nurse invited me to take part in a medical mission trip to Ecuador. We would be away for a week and staying in Quito, Ecuador. I volunteered to see as many children as I could in that week: examine them and treat them with whatever remedy I saw fit.

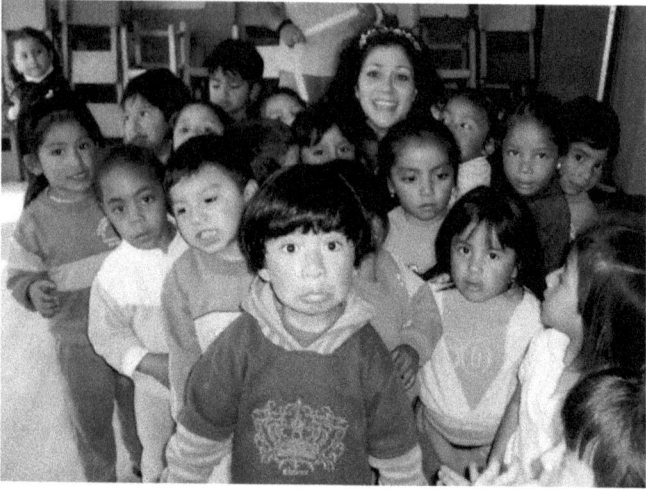

That week away was a beautiful experience. Being away from my family and the United States and seeing the poverty that is there and how happy and grateful people are in spite of their circumstances, really hit home with me. It made me grateful for what I had and at the same time inspired me to make the best of my situation.

My husband picked me up at the airport upon my return from Ecuador. When I saw our house as he drove us up the driveway, I turned to him and said, "I have had this week to think things over, and I don't see how we can continue to live emotionally disconnected the rest of our lives." I saw no other choice but to ask him for a divorce to free myself from a loveless marriage.

He agreed that neither of us had been truly happy with each other. We apologized to each other for not creating the life together that each of us thought we wanted, recognizing that we were emotionally disconnected from each other. He was okay with my decision; it didn't bother him as much as it bothered me.

What bothered me the most was that I wanted to have an emotional connection with a man, and I wanted to create a loving experience. I just couldn't see myself continuing to live in that situation because I knew that there could be something else, something much deeper.

I was hopeful I would meet someone else in the future and create a loving marriage. I grew up with loving grandparents and in a loving family environment. I had also seen many loving and happy family relationships in my office. That's what I wanted for myself.

We went ahead with the divorce. After we got divorced, I found myself physically alone after I purchased my own house. In the office, I was financially alone, without the support of a partner. Shortly after, my oldest daughter started college, so I had that financial burden as well. I realized it was all on my shoulders to create the life I wanted.

It was up to me to meet a man with whom I could build a mutually loving relationship. It was up to me to create a career with a solid financial future that would provide for my two daughters and me.

That is why I started searching the Internet and listening to podcasts and YouTube videos for inspiration and ideas. And that is when I discovered the teachings of Louise Hay, Wayne Dyer, Abraham Hicks, Derek Rydall, Christie Marie Sheldon, Joe Dispenza, Marc Allen, Marissa Peers, Marianne Williamson, and my mentor Gina Devee (Divine Living Academy), to name a few.

Listening to all their talks and podcasts, I learned about not letting life happen to you, but choosing instead to create your own life with your imagination. That is how I transitioned from the office. I started imagining an office that was overflowing with patients and that was abundantly supporting me financially.

I started doing extra work outside of the area as a hospitalist. I visualized myself going to the local hospital. I would eventually end up closing my own office and becoming a full-time hospitalist.

First, I visualized myself going to the hospital only—no longer going to the office because the hospital was a much better opportunity for me to serve more patients. At the same time, a hospital setting would free up more of my time because I would have set hours; I would not be the sole person on-call like I was with my patients in the office. Instead, I would take turns with other physicians.

Financially, it was a much more beneficial opportunity for me. I used the law of attraction to imagine my new job status. The opportunity came after imagining it for several months. All of a sudden, I got a phone call from one of the hospital administrators that a children's hospital was hiring hospitalists to take care of children and wanted me to contract with them. I jumped at the opportunity because this was what I had been wishing for. That was how I transitioned from office work to hospital work.

THE OFFICE

During my divorce, while I was imagining transitioning to a hospitalist role, not only was I seeing the association between my emotions—how I got sick every time I felt sad—I also started seeing associations in the children and the families who were coming into the office.

There were many families who were happier and more prosperous than others, and they seemed to have more opportunities, more ideas, and more of a positive mindset. I discovered that they were eating healthier because they were consuming more fruits and vegetables and more water. Additionally, these families were typically only coming in once a year for their children's physicals.

Mindset and Emotions Connection

The families that were struggling financially were primarily eating fast foods or school lunches. The parents were much less actively involved in what the children were eating or not eating. The children were often not getting meals prepared at home. Additionally, they had a fatalistic mindset, in other words: whatever happens, happens.

Parents were often smokers, and their children would get frequent colds. I would inform parents about the studies showing children who are exposed to second-hand smoke get five times more colds per year than children who are not exposed. As I said, these parents either had a fatalistic idea of their health, or they were not actively involved in maintaining their own standard of health, which included not exercising, smoking, and/or eating processed foods.

Children who do not take part in regular physical activities and who are living on a diet that is high in fast foods and junk foods may suffer with frequent upper respiratory infections and have a greater chance of being obese. There is definitely a connection.

I saw this pattern repeat itself as the years passed in the office setting. I examined this pattern more closely. During conversations with children or their parents, I started to make the connection between a child's emotions and the specific parts of the body they were experiencing issues with, or the reasons for their office visit.

For example, when parents would share with me thoughts about being stuck with past influences, of not being able to move forward, or of not having any positive ideas or hope for the future—in other words parents who had that kind of stagnant energy—I noticed their children were having symptoms of constipation. Constipation is a physical ailment that is associated with that type of stuck energy and negative emotion of hopelessness.

Later in the chapter, I will be sharing the following with you:

- A list of emotional ailments
- The negative emotion that is associated with the ailment
- A positive affirmation to help you transform the ailment

I also list natural remedies that you can use at the same time to support you, physically and emotionally, to overcome all types of health issues.

Figuring Out a Solution

I wanted to help my patients. I tried a positive affirmation. That was my way of trying to figure out the solution.

> *If X disease was associated with X negative emotion, then I am going to find X positive emotion or affirmation to help the person transition from that negative mindset.*

I don't want people to think they need to force themselves to become positive and happy; that's not what I'm talking about. It's about recognizing that negative thoughts are making you sick. There is a definite association between the energetic vibration of your thoughts and how your body is responding to them.

I'm suggesting that improvement in a particular ailment can be experienced with some kind of affirmation that you repeat so your body experiences the different energy required for a particular organ system to heal.

> *The mind is everything.*
> *What you think, you become.*
> ~ attributed to Buddha

Affirmations Are the Connections Between Diseases and Emotions

In my search for answers through readings, research, and many conferences I attended, I considered my own personal health issues, and wanted to help my patients and their families in the office. I realized that a lot of things are based on the number three. The number three is considered Divinity.

I believe our bodies are made up of our mental emotions, our physical bodies, and our spirit or our soul.

My method of treating patients, my family, and myself is to approach every physical ailment from those three dimensions:

- To use *natural remedies* to treat the physical body
- To use *positive affirmations* to treat the mind and emotions

- To use *prayer and meditation* to soothe or to support our spirit and our soul

Incorporating these three modalities, I believe a person can experience true health. Our bodies are meant to be healthy all the time. We are not meant to be sad. We are not meant to be frustrated. We are not meant to have physical pain.

We are meant to have a spiritual connection.

All three dimensions must be nurtured, cared for, and supported for us to have true health.

Free will is a major implication. If you don't take part in actively thinking about what you're eating, what you're drinking, what you're putting into your body, then your physical body is not well taken care of. God and the Universe won't intervene because of free will; the mistreatment will continue as long as you allow it to continue.

If your body, mind, emotions, and spirit are all supported with like-minded individuals, meditation, and energy healing, it is easy to feel like a weight has been lifted from your shoulders because all things are working with each other. Ultimately, that is what everyone is looking for. We want to be loved and healthy, and we are looking to find purpose, meaning, and a connection with the Universe.

THE RESULTS

Below is a list of the health ailments, the emotions that could have led to that ailment, and an affirmation or inspirational thought. I'd also like to offer you a list of natural remedies that can support and ameliorate your physical illness so there is truly a combination of body, mind, and spirit to help you and your children find natural solutions to many common health ailments.

Emotion/ Negative Thought	Body Part/Health Issue	Affirmation, Meditation
Any fear, feeling stuck, holding on to repressed or immobilized feelings, pulling away, escaping, retreating, running away.	Hyperactivity, biting, abdominal cramps, constipation, excessive appetite or loss of appetite, gastritis, bowel problems, diarrhea, heartburn, indigestion, Crohn's disease, ulcerative colitis, nausea, hyperventilation, asthma, emphysema, pneumonia, bronchitis, snoring, skin problems, hives, urticaria, edema, swellings, fistula, chills, body odors, fainting, dizziness, headaches, coma, car sickness, anemia, leg problems, corns, low back pain, foot problems, joint problems, vision problems, eye problems, hemorrhoids, menopausal problems, sterility, miscarriage.	I am safe and I am loved; I approve of myself. I am at peace with my past. I am free to create a life that I love. I am safe to choose my life freely. I am creating a life of freedom and joy. I love myself, I love you, I love my child, I love others. You are loved, you are safe, you are my precious child. You are a precious gift, a part of the Universe, God, Allah, Spirit, Divinity (choose your own word that applies to your belief here).

Emotion/ Negative Thought	Body Part/Health Issue	*Affirmation, Meditation*
		I am, have, and create love and joy in my life. Every day I am doing/will do something good for myself to move me forward. My dreams are step by step coming closer every day. Miracles happen every day and I accept a Divine healing for myself or my child. And so it is! (In Jesus' name). *If it applies to your beliefs, repeat:* World without end! Amen. All is well in my/ my child's future.

Emotion/ Negative Thought	Body Part/Health Issue	Affirmation, Meditation, Prayer
Sad, unhappy, joyless, hopeless, unloved, unheard, down, rejected, lonely, disconnected from the world or others, defenseless, pointless, thoughtless, no motivation, no aspirations or goals, trapped, imprisoned, victimized, stressed out, repressed anger, procrastinating, burdened, overwhelmed, unsupported.	Depression, cystic fibrosis, cysts, abscesses, deafness, fatigue, insomnia, sleep problems, post-nasal drip, suicidal, excessive crying, edema, congestive heart failure, heart attacks, genital male-female identity issues, relationship problems, divorce, joint aches and pains, premature aging, Alzheimer's, dementia, hair loss, weight gain, obesity, immobility, hernias, hypoglycemia, hypothermia, hypothyroidism, gray hairs, incontinence, impotence, lupus, palsies.	Life loves me; I love and approve of myself. I am at peace with and forgive all my emotions. I choose to take in life fully, freely and easily. I am enthusiastic about life and filled with energy. I create and am in control of my own destiny/ future. I am creating a peaceful, loving, and joyful life for myself and my children. I love and approve of myself/ my child, and others love and approve of me. I create a new life with new rules that totally support me and my children.

Emotion/ Negative Thought	Body Part/Health Issue	Affirmation, Meditation, Prayer
Anger, anxiety, frustration, bitterness, resentful, hatred, punishment, raging, violent, refusing, rejecting, revenge-seeking, denial, anxiety, nonaccepting, domineering, blaming, stressed out, nervous, anguish, stubbornness, critical.	Cuts, depression, fever, nail-biting, nervousness, coughing, dysmenorrhea, body image or self-image problems, self-hurting, earaches, eye problems, boils, cellulite, carpal tunnel syndrome, eczema, epilepsy, seizures, obesity, overweight, bleeding (note where), female and male self-problems, impotence, goiter, gallstones, gout, halitosis, canker sores, bursitis, burns, premature aging, Alzheimer's, dementia, all inflammation and -itis ailments, jaundice, liver problems, nodules, tumors, neuralgias, neck problems, kidney problems, kidney stones.	I create a life filled with love, light, and rewards. I am at peace with myself. I accept and forgive myself. I am at peace with others, the world, Universe, Divinity. The world/Universe supports me/is on my side and helps me every day. I am creating/ will create a peaceful, supportive life for myself with ease and joy. I am creating/ will create only loving experiences in my joyful world. I am creating a loving family. I choose to be at peace in my life.

Emotion/ Negative Thought	Body Part/Health Issue	Affirmation, Meditation, Prayer
		I have love, compassion, and tolerance for myself, my child, and others. Love, peace, and joy are what I know. I look for love and find it everywhere

FAQs

1. *What is your Favorite Affirmation of all or go-to one for most problems?*

   My go-to is: I am willing to change the patterns in me that created this (fill in the blank) condition. I love and approve of myself (or others, if relationship issue). I am safe to create new thought patterns that will support and help heal me.

2. *Where and how often do you do this?*

   My favorite location is anywhere you are alone (as a mom, even while brushing my teeth or showering!).

Preferably more than once a day, mornings and evenings, in a comfortable quiet place. I also like to rub on or diffuse the essential oil most appropriate for X condition while chanting.

3. *What do you recommend to say at the end or conclude with?*

I like to say: "And so it is!" Also "in Jesus' name" or just Amen or Namaste, whatever empowers and feels good to you is fine.

Natural Remedies for Your Body

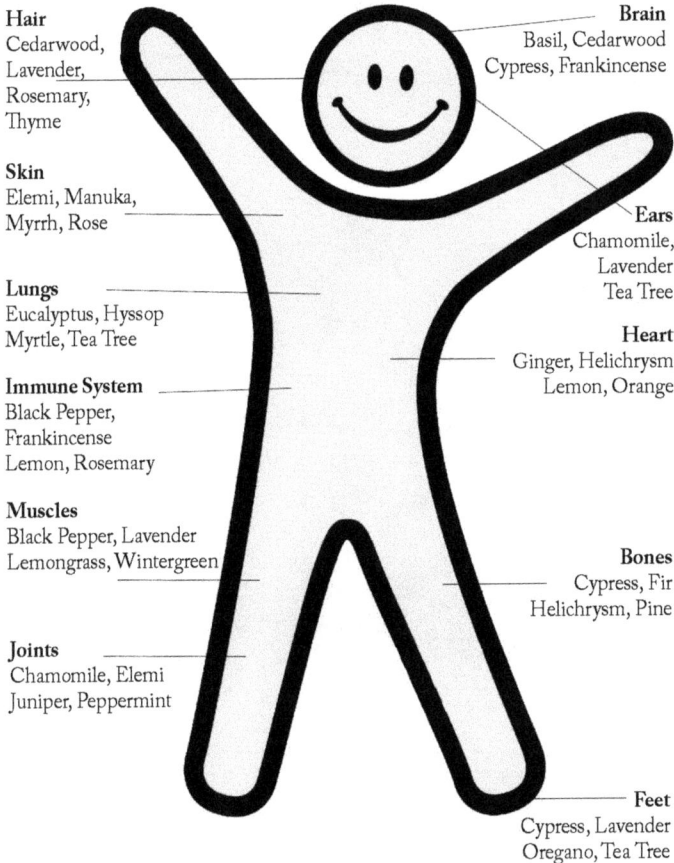

Hair
Cedarwood,
Lavender,
Rosemary,
Thyme

Skin
Elemi, Manuka,
Myrrh, Rose

Lungs
Eucalyptus, Hyssop
Myrtle, Tea Tree

Immune System
Black Pepper,
Frankincense
Lemon, Rosemary

Muscles
Black Pepper, Lavender
Lemongrass, Wintergreen

Joints
Chamomile, Elemi
Juniper, Peppermint

Brain
Basil, Cedarwood
Cypress, Frankincense

Ears
Chamomile,
Lavender
Tea Tree

Heart
Ginger, Helichrysm
Lemon, Orange

Bones
Cypress, Fir
Helichrysm, Pine

Feet
Cypress, Lavender
Oregano, Tea Tree

CHAPTER THREE

Body, Mind, and Spirit

Do you not know that your bodies are temples of the Holy Spirit who is in you, whom you have received from God? . . . Therefore honor God with your bodies.
1 Corinthians 6:19–20, NIV

Body, mind, and spirit are the three components to your health. The above passage from the Bible is a reminder that you are in control of your health. The components of health are our body and self-image, our mind and emotions, and our spirit or soul. These three components are connected to each other, and how they play and contribute to each other affect our overall health.

YOUR BODY AND SELF-IMAGE

Your body and self-image contribute to your emotions, which contribute to your diseases. The way you feel about your body creates energy inside your body, which is related to and contributes to your emotions.

Over the years in my practice and as a hospitalist, I have noticed that patients were coming in with certain complaints about their bodies and certain diseases. They all seemed to have a grouping of emotions that correlated with that problem body part. For example, digestive problems are associated with emotions of having trouble accepting and processing an aspect of your life, of your current life situation. I noticed a correlation with that.

Feelings and emotions about the body cause certain emotional ideas in your mind to occur and vice versa. These can include, for example, fear or sadness or resentment. Those are associated with certain ailments and certain body parts being affected.

My Patients

Throughout my time as a practitioner and during my hospital work, I noticed that patients were coming in with the same ailments. I was able to associate those ailments with certain emotions. For example, there are a lot of diseases and body ailments that are associated with fear, which I listed in the previous chapter. Fear, anxiety, refusal to let go, any type of stuck feeling—I noticed that these were associated with certain diseases like gastrointestinal problems, skin problems, breathing issues, and major organ systems being affected.

As I noted in the previous chapter, the ailments that are mostly associated with fear, which occurred with me as well, center around an emotional trauma—holding on to the past in frustration. I noticed in these instances that my immune system was weakened. If I continued to think about a previous problem, it would inevitably lead to my health deteriorating for a few days after that time.

I am putting together a list of the opposite to the emotion or fear that caused this disease problem.

The Solution: Affirmations

I wrote a list of affirmations and positive ideas and thoughts that I could turn to whenever I had a negative thought pattern. I created the affirmations to reverse or tune in to the opposite of the negative thought while making them realistic and keeping them in the present as if it is already true.

I came up with the idea of having a positive affirmation, like: *I am looking forward to the future,* and I assigned it an opposite thought or emotion to transform the negative thought. Every time I would have a negative thought and I felt myself deteriorating, I would counteract it with a positive affirmation.

For example, if the fear of the future came up, which is highly associated with leg problems because our legs are what move us forward, I would recite the positive affirmation mentioned above: *I am looking forward to the future; I move forward with confidence and joy.* These affirmations were a way for me to help myself change my mind and my thoughts of the current problem.

I repeated them at least twice a day, together with using other natural therapies. This helped me greatly through the years, and the patients I saw in the office and in the hospital experienced changes and success using these protocols as well.

I also recommend nutritional and exercise support along with the affirmations and the natural remedies. Look at what you're putting in your body, but also what you're putting *on* it, and what it is exposed to. To address health issues, we can add natural remedies to help us feel better, but we also need to take away any toxins that interrupt our well-being.

YOUR MIND

In this next section, we will be examining the mind. Your mind is powerful.

How My Mind and Thoughts Led to Emotions and Diseases

I noticed over the years that when my mind would whirl with negative ideas and feelings and moods due to my external world, my health was affected by these negative patterns. For example, if I had a rough day at work, I would come home and feel really tired. Then I would start thinking about someone who had upset me or a situation that had bothered me during the day. Inevitably, these thoughts and feelings would lead to either illness or some part of my body experiencing pain. I noticed that same association with the patients in the office.

Our emotions and thoughts are stored energy that correlates to certain parts of our bodies. We react to these emotions in one of two ways. Stored energy from positive thoughts and emotions tends to leave us feeling healthy. However, stored energy from negative thoughts and emotions often leads to a breakdown of one of these components, which then leads to health issues or the breakdown of the function of one of the organ systems, typically corresponding with the specific emotion that is occurring.

My Patients' Experiences

In the office and in the hospital, I learned so much from my patients. For example, many children would come in with throat problems, such as a sore throat or hoarseness, and I noticed that often the throat problems were associated with fear of speaking up, not being allowed to express themselves, or feeling that what they said did not matter. They were either mad because they couldn't speak, afraid to speak, or resentful that someone told them not to speak. This is a perfect example of an association of the negative emotion and how a body part is affected.

Hearing problems are associated with something a child should have heard, didn't want to hear, or didn't hear.

It's the same with the eyes:

- What are they supposed to see that they are not seeing? What did they see that they did not have to or want to see?

- What is occurring in their life that they may not have intellectually conceptualized yet? Or what have they intellectualized only with child-like understanding, misunderstanding, or only at a subconscious level?

Sometimes we are not intellectually aware of the emotion causing the body's health issue.

The Solution: Affirmations

The solution occurred to me after seeing this pattern in so many patients and myself.

When I have a negative emotion or health issue, what is the opposite emotion that I can create an affirmation about to turn it into a positive light—something hopeful, something that will move me forward?

That is how I came up with the positive affirmations listed in Chapter Two. They keep your mind from focusing on what you don't want, they move you forward, and instead, you're focusing on the change you want to occur. (See the chart at the end of Chapter Two for examples.)

YOUR SPIRIT

> *I pray that all may go well with you and*
> *that you may be in good health,*
> *as it goes well with your soul.*
>
> 3 John 1:2, ESV

Our spirit or our soul can also lead to emotions and diseases because this is our connection with Divinity or the Universe. Also, it is our grounding with Mother Earth. And it also correlates with our core idea of our self, our connection to our higher self, our gut, or that little voice inside.

Keeping my spirit healthy is important to me, and it's an important message to share with others to help them stay healthy.

If we are not connected to the earth, if we don't feel a connection with Divinity, if we don't have a sense of our higher self, if we are not listening to that inner voice, a disconnect occurs for our spirituality and a breakdown within the three components of our health occurs. It's like a domino effect. If any of these three deteriorate or are negatively traumatized in any way, then it affects our overall health.

Taking Care of Your Body, Mind, and Spirit

Because your health is made up of these three components, the way to take care of them is to be aware of what you put in and what comes out of your body.

Your diet, the nutrition your body is receiving, and the medications your body is receiving are examples of what you put in your body. Over the years, I have seen significant health improvements in my patients who ate organically and mainly fruits and vegetables. There are several studies that have been done over many years that show the benefits of eating whole foods, taking organic supplements, and limiting the amount of food that you take in.

Another way to help take care of your body is exercise. Our bodies are meant to move every day. We are not meant to be sedentary. If you are sitting in a chair at a desk for eight hours a day, you need to make the extra effort of moving your body periodically, even if it means doing jumping jacks at your desk or taking the stairs instead of the elevator.

Our bodies were made to walk, to move all day long. Scheduling at least half an hour of exercise, three days a week, is important, especially to the bones, joints, and muscles in your body. Or, my favorite: park your car in the lot as far away as possible from the building you're entering to make yourself walk the extra steps. Every bit adds up every day!

I also want to talk about products we put on our bodies and the ingredients these products contain. There has been much research done on toxic ingredients, and currently there are still a lot of toxic ingredients in every product we physically put on our bodies. Consider not only lotions and shampoos, but also the products we use to maintain our homes—

household cleaning products that we touch and inhale, such as aerosols and sprays.

Additionally, as you know, there are a lot of toxic ingredients in cigarette smoke, which can affect you even when you are not the one smoking the cigarettes.

To be proactive, we must be increasingly aware of the toxic ingredients that are approved for use in manufacturing, in spite of being harmful to our health. A perfect example of this is paraben. *Parabens* are used as preservatives in products such as body lotions, shampoos, and body-care products. Parabens have been outlawed in all of Europe, yet are still widely used in manufacturing in the United States.

Next are OTC and prescription medications. Even if we are healthy, most of us need to use medicine at one time or another, even if it is just for a cut. Be mindful of the products you are putting in or on your body, the side effects they are known to cause, and the toxic ingredients that may be in the products, causing a negative side effect.

I have witnessed the side effects of some of the ingredients of nonnatural or artificially made medications. It's almost like playing Russian roulette.

Are you going to be the one that is going to get the negative side effect that is warned about on the package, or will it be your child?

Every single man-made medication has a negative side effect. There are no prescribed or OTC man-made products that I know of that do not list a potential negative side effect. I'm sure you've seen commercials on TV where the announcer quickly lists the potential side effects of the drug they have just promoted as being the answer to your problem. Some of the potential side effects are quite serious. Please also read *all* of your medication labels closely and their package insert lists of side effects.

It really hit home with me as a physician who prescribes medications every single day. I vowed a Hippocratic Oath to do no harm. The thought that I was prescribing something that could potentially cause serious side effects for my patients turned my world upside down; that is why I turned to searching for and recommending natural remedies.

In my experience, most natural, organic, plant-based remedies have far fewer negative effects than pharmaceuticals when taken appropriately with the guidance of an experienced holistic practitioner. They are much purer and safer, and contain no, or very small amounts, of preservatives or toxic ingredients. Over the past several years, many research studies have been published about the benefits of whole food nutrition and organic, plant-based remedies. There are evidence-based, double-blind, placebo-controlled studies that confirm these claims.

Additionally, there are published and well-known studies that have specifically tested one natural remedy against a disease process, for example, Echinacea. Studies revealed that Echinacea helps boost the immune system and reduces the number of days that a person is sick from a common cold by 26 percent.[1] This may not seem significant, but it's a huge start toward confirming the efficacy of a natural remedy. To name a few, frankincense and turmeric have been studied as anti-inflammatories; lavender has also been studied as a natural remedy for several sleep issues.

And much more research is under way currently for new therapies, such as:

- DNA repair and gene editing technology
- Nutrigenomics
- Organic electronics
- Synthetic biology
- Bioidentical implants
- Redox signaling molecules
- Robotic surgery
- Music and energy healing
- Virtual and 3-D medicine[2]

---

1 Watson, Leon. "Largest ever clinical study into echinacea finds herbal remedy CAN protect against colds." 10 Oct 2012. Dailymail.com/Health
2 Ellis, Monique. "Technologies of 2019." proclinical.com; Nwazor, Toby. "Five emerging technologies in science that will shape our lives in the coming years." huffpost.com

My mission is now to discover more about how I can combine natural remedies with positive affirmations to help alleviate health issues for my patients, my family, and myself.

In conclusion, if any part of your system is off balance—whether it's an organ system, an emotion, or your spiritual being, there will be a ripple effect, which ultimately will affect your entire body system and lead to health issues, diseases, or a breakdown of functions that will eventually lead to diseases.

There are simple, natural, easy to use options to maintain or regain your health. You simply need to consistently use them and believe in them. Take back control of your health by connecting with your body, improving your mindset, allowing yourself to be guided by your soul, and working with a licensed naturopath or holistic healthcare provider.

CHAPTER FOUR

Products and Medicines: Toxicity and Side Effects

TOXICITY AND TOXIC INGREDIENTS

As mentioned, it isn't merely foods and medicines with toxic, man-made, artificial ingredients—including preservatives, fillers, and nonorganic contaminants such as hormones and pesticides—that we take internally that cause us harm, it's also the products we use on our skin and the toxins we breathe in from the air. I highly recommend that you become aware of the ingredients in everything that you use and expose your children and yourself to; read the ingredients in everything you put on your body, in your body, and breathe into your lungs.

Toxic Ingredients and Their Effects

During my years of transitioning to alternative medicine, I became aware that many ingredients that are widely used in the United States have been outright outlawed or increased sanctions have been placed on them in other countries.

I have been blessed to travel to Europe several times. During my visits, I learned that more than 1300 chemicals are currently banned in all European countries compared to only 30 in the U.S.A. Parabens, for example, have been outlawed in all European countries since around 2014. Parabens are an ingredient that is in most of the body lotions and hair-care products available in the United States. Research since 2011 shows BPA and paraben are toxic substances that are associated with hormonal changes in the body. It specifically turns into estrogen in the body, and this estrogen is bound by fat cells.[3] The study also showed that paraben blocked the effectiveness of cancer drugs, like Tamoxifen.

Ingredients that affect our hormones that are absorbed into fat cells are associated with a theory of why some people have trouble losing weight. The theory is that your fat cells have stored the toxic ingredients from your use of these products, making it difficult to lose weight. It isn't just a hormonal change that the toxic ingredients cause—like mood swings and emotional problems—they also affect your fat cells, which can negatively impact your weight loss efforts.

---

3 Colliver, Victoria. "BPA, methylparaben, block breast cancer drugs" Calif. Pacific Medical Center, SF. Sept, 2011. sfgate.com; "Methylparaben Human Health Effects: Toxicity Summary." toxnet. nlm.nih.gov

In 2001, DDT, which is a pesticide, was banned from worldwide use,[4] except in certain areas of Africa where they still need it to combat malaria. All the countries that have banned DDT have come up with new chemical pesticides that are organic and natural and that are as effective; they simply don't have high levels of toxicity.

> New chemical pesticides have been created to replace DDT with safe levels of toxicity, approved by the EPA, and then monitored by the FDA. DDT has been associated with everything from skin irritation, nausea, and headaches, to hormonal or reproductive disorders, autism, and possibly cancer.[5]

Mutagenesis is a "method of plant breeding that involves exposing plants to radiation or chemicals in a way that scrambles their genes in order to produce a new trait or more plants."[6]

In an article, "No Turtles Here, Just Mutated Food," Nick Meyer states the Organic Consumers' Association proposes mutagenesis can cause unknown toxins or allergens when we are exposed to these mutated food products. The main food groups that are being grown using mutagenesis are barley,

---

4 epa.gov
5 Chavez, Obeydah. "Pesticides: Harmful Effects on Human Health." *Liberty Voice.* 27 June 2014. guardianlv.com/2014/06/pesticides-harmful-effects-on-human-health
6 "Tell the USDA National Organic Program: Mutagenesis Doesn't Belong in Organic!" *Organic Consumers Association.* organicconsumers. org/action_archive/action-13727.html?action_key=13727

cotton, grapefruit, pears, rice, sunflowers, wheat, soy, and corn.[7]

TOXIC INGREDIENTS[8]

Hair

- *Shampoos and Conditioners*: fragrance, paraben, phthalates, petrolatum, propylene glycol, SLS, SLES
- *Color/Dyes*: synthetic colors (FD&D or D&C), toluene, formaldehyde, hydrogen peroxide
- *Spray, Gels, Balms*: fragrance, petrolatum, paraben, propylene glycol

Face

- *Lotions, Moisturizers, Scar and Antiwrinkle Creams*: See *skin*.
- *Makeup*: titanium, heavy metals, petrolatum, synthetic colors and dyes, tar, formaldehyde

---

7 Meyer, Nick. "No Turtles Here, Just Mutated Food: Here Are 7 Crops Being Grown with Mutated Seeds." *AltHealth Works*. 07 July 2017. althealthworks.com/3568/no-turtles-here-just-mutated-food-here-are-7-food-crops-being-grown-from-mutated-seeds-seriously
8 Some information in this list was taken from: Alvi, Saniya. "10 Beauty Product Ingredients You Definitely Want to Avoid." www.healthprep.com

Mouth

- *Food*: pesticides, insecticides, hormones, preservatives, food coloring and dyes
- *Water*: BPA, pesticides, bacteria, ova, parasites, fungi, larva
- *Toothpaste*: SLS, hydrogen peroxide

Underarm

- *Anti-perspirants and Deodorants*: aluminum, formaldehyde, titanium dioxide, other metals

Nails

- *Nail Polish:* formaldehyde, toluene, alcohol

Genitalia

- *Talc*: asbestos
- *Creams and Lotions*: See *skin*
- *Tampons and Pads*: dioxins, furams (from chlorine), pesticide residues from cotton, fragrance chemicals

Skin

- *Lotions, Creams, Moisturizers, Sunblock/Sunscreens, Cleaning Products*: fragrance chemicals, chlorine, formaldehyde, propylene glycol, paraben, phthalates, petrolatum, mineral oil, oxybenzone, triclosan, salicylates (aspirin), SLS, SLES, alcohol

For more information or to order clean products, go to: www.purehaven.com/drruth

Searching for Choices and Solutions

As I searched for a solution to replace the products that I was using and putting into my body, I attended several conferences, researched and read widely, and asked authority figures in the area. I concluded that we do have a choice. There are many options available.

Eating organic is one very helpful choice. Farmers and product manufacturers must comply and go out of their way to become organic. These products are much better choices to take care of my patients' and my own health, choices that ensure we don't take in harmful toxic ingredients or have to worry about their harmful effects.

I recommend all my patients and clients eat organic foods as much as possible and to use natural, nontoxic, preservative-free products. I encourage them to avoid pesticides for gardening, and, as much as possible, to read the labels and ingredients to create a toxin-free environment.

NEGATIVE SIDE EFFECTS

I want to make the reader aware that even if you don't know that you're taking something that has a toxic ingredient in it, typically man-made medicine or drugs will cause a negative side effect.

Awareness and Labels

I am increasingly aware of labels every day as a physician when I look at every single drug that I prescribe, whether it is a prescription or an OTC drug. When you look at them, if they are man-made, they most likely have a list of negative side effects. The label may list something as mild as a skin irritation or something as drastic as suicide ideations, or sudden death.

When you receive the insert with your prescribed medication from the pharmacy, be aware and proactive and read it to discover potential side effects. Ask your physician—as he or she is looking up the medication to prescribe in the reference book, which is about three inches thick—for the list of every single potential side effect.

There are no prescription or over-the-counter (OTC) nonorganic medications that I have seen in twenty-four years of being a pediatrician that do not have a list of side effects. Even if you don't know the toxic ingredients you are taking, you may experience some side effect, minor or otherwise. It could be not being able to lose weight, sleep issues, headache, or irritability.

Most likely, particularly with long-term use of toxic medications, a side effect ultimately occurs. It is very rare not to experience a negative side effect. What a disservice we are doing to our children by putting them on long-term medications that can give them a side effect now or years in the future.

Wanting to Cause No Harm

Almost every day in the office, I would see patients who came in with a physical or emotional complaint that was later revealed to be related to prescribed medications the child was taking. When I reviewed the history and the medications prescribed to the child, I increasingly became aware of the connection.

For example, a particular medication had a listed side effect of headaches. The parents didn't know nor did they read the information sheet from the pharmacy that headaches were a probable side effect of the medication. I felt terrible as a human, as a mother, and especially as the physician that was prescribing the medication. I was the probable cause of this child's negative side effect. By trying to help him with his current illness, I was inadvertently creating another problem.

What a disservice we are doing to our patients and children by giving them a second medication, which I often see happen. Physicians are prescribing a second medication to alleviate the side effect of the first medication. It made me think about my role in this situation and what more we have to learn in the healthcare industry.

During the last few years, I have incorporated the spiritual and emotional side of diseases. With the thousands of families I have seen go through my office and those I have attended to in my hospital work, I have learned how a child's emotions, which are related to their current experiences or what is happening in the family dynamic, can make them feel or not feel and how that is associated with their disease process.

I want to pass the baton. I don't want to be the gatekeeper; I am just a helper for the parents. I don't want to make you feel like you are solely responsible. I want you to see that it is a partnership between yourself and your healthcare worker in proactively taking care of your child's and your own health.

It needs to be less about you visiting your doctor and saying: *Here is my child's problem. What is your solution, doctor?* I want people to feel some sense of accountability, to be proactive. You do have choices and options.

It is more than just what your doctor is suggesting for you to take or avoid at that moment. It is also looking at everything that is involved with the disease, including the emotional part, and the physical part so you are aware of the mind, body, and spirit working together that ultimately created the disease.

Together with your healthcare advocate, you can find a solution, working with the mind, body, and spirit to help eliminate the health problem that you or your child may be experiencing.

NATURAL PRODUCTS

As a way to encourage a lifestyle change, I like to promote natural products and at the same time educate my patients on their efficacy. This includes both natural medicines for ailments and natural products for everyday use to help their bodies heal themselves.

My goal is to help patients create a lifestyle change involving their mind, body, and spirit with natural products so they don't have to worry about negative side effects or toxic ingredient when choosing the natural medicine or product that will be the most effective for them.

As mentioned, the effectiveness of natural medicine has been proven in the research, articles, and patient care protocols that have emerged within the past five years. We are living in a time of medicine revolution and we are just at the beginning of using natural medicines for everything healthcare related.

Last year, close to 40,000 people attended an essential oil conference in Salt Lake City, Utah.[9] Fifty-one thousand people ran the New York City Marathon, and close to 10,000 attended an Organic Nutritional Product convention in Florida.[10] We are becoming increasingly oriented to plant-based remedies, such as essential oils as an option for our healthcare and we are recognizing that exercise is a significant factor for improving our body's health, as well as how it positively affects our emotions.

Meditation and mindfulness are being exponentially used in schools, in hospitals, in training groups, in conferences, and even in traditional Western medicine realms. Meditation and mindfulness are being included in practices because we are becoming increasingly aware of the benefits of integrating them with exercise and natural products into our lifestyle to improve all aspects of our health.

How Natural Products Work

The difference of how your body reacts to a natural versus a non-natural product is as follows. A non-natural product is specifically designed to give your body the message for the ailment you are attempting to treat.

For example, an antibiotic is killing bacteria in your body. It's an external force that is put inside your body that tells your

9 mydoterra.com/ruthrodriguez3
10 juiceplus.com/+ruthrodriguez

body what to do. Your body has no choice because it is forced to act in a certain way due to the medication you have taken. Your body must succumb to what the product is telling it to do or what the product is doing to it.

When we use a natural product, the plant-based product supports that organ system for the part of your body that you are treating. Your body recognizes it as natural. It is not going to have to process it. Your body simply absorbs it and lets it help that organ system heal without having a side effect because your body recognizes the product.

Then, your liver and your kidneys don't have to be affected because the cells recognize the product as natural. It is absorbed naturally.

No Toxic Ingredients or Negative Side Effects

The reason your body recognizes a product as natural is because it comes from a plant. It is absorbed and processed without creating a negative side effect. It is simply helping your body do what it naturally does.

A human body is an incredible machine that heals itself. Taking a natural product is giving your body the nutrients or the amino acids or the enzymes that it needs to heal that disease process. Your body wants to be healthy. Its natural state is to be perfectly healthy, not to be diseased.

By giving it a natural substance, you are helping it do just that. You are giving your body the substrate that aids in making it healthy again. That is why there are no toxic effects. With a natural product, your body doesn't have to process anything like it does with a man-made product in order to turn it into another chemical so your body can eliminate it. It doesn't have to send it to fat cells to be stored. It doesn't have to succumb to the side effect caused by the non-natural substance.

Effectiveness

The effectiveness of natural medicine and products is giving your body the substrates, the enzymes, the nutrients, the amino acids, and the chemicals that it needs for the body to heal itself. That is where the effectiveness of natural medicine comes in.

Over the years, I have learned that many products in natural medicine can be used for multiple health ailments; this has been an interesting paradigm shift for me. It's been a reassurance that I can treat someone with lavender oil for a headache, a skin rash, or sleep problems.

If the lavender oil happens not to have worked for the particular problem I'm treating, there is always another natural product or medicine that I could prescribe instead. There are so many products that treat multiple health issues and vice versa, multiple health issues can be treated with a variety of natural products.

There are many more choices with natural medicine. In traditional Western medicine, in my experience, the options to treat your allergy problems, for example, are limited. This is especially true in pediatrics; there are fewer options because of the age constrictions.

I cannot prescribe the same medications to a six-month-old baby that I can to a three-year-old child because products don't have FDA approval, or research has not been conducted for children under two. And, there may only be one or two choices of medicines to prescribe for a three-year-old child suffering with allergies.

In the natural medicine world, I can think of five different natural remedies that will work for a three-year-old child with allergies. That has been enlightening to have so many tools in my pockets. Natural medicine protocols are filled with solutions to help my patients, while in Western medicine, I felt I was restricted to very few possibilities. The world of health has opened for me.

If someone said: *I don't want to take anything that is plant-based. I only want to take a prescription medication because I want it to be FDA-approved,* I could still offer them a natural remedy in combination with the FDA-approved medication.

I would give them their FDA-approved prescription because that is their mindset, it will make them happy, and that is what they believe will work for them. But I can also suggest to them other alternative therapies and natural remedies to help with the specific health ailment.

It is much more of a collaborative, integrated effort where the patient benefits much more and helps themselves versus my helping them solely with traditional Western methods.

CHAPTER FIVE

Encouragement and Empowerment

GETTING YOUR CHILD HEALTHY WITH NATURAL PRODUCTS

I would like to empower you by letting you know that there are many resources out there. If you take it upon yourself or seek help from others, please understand that we really are in a state of change in medicine where natural therapies are going to become more and more our standard way of care.

I want to empower you to feel and believe it is possible to heal your child and to improve the overall health of every member of your family using solely natural plant-based products and nutrition.

Awareness of the Problem

In my journey as a physician, I was blessed to become increasingly aware of all the toxic ingredients and negative side effects of everything that I was prescribing to my patients. My close communication with the families in my office and in the hospital, my research into the ingredients found in Western medicine, and the feedback I was getting from the patients gave me this awareness.

As an individual, you might be saying to yourself: *I am not medically trained, so how am I going to know if there is a problem with what I'm taking already, even when it has been prescribed by a licensed physician?*

I want to help you become aware of this by recommending you look at the ingredients, the potential side effects of those ingredients, and what toxicities may occur in your body by taking in these ingredients. In medical school, traditional doctors, myself included, do not receive extra instruction on the real consequences of man-made ingredients, some of which are fillers or added to make a product taste better.

There are many ingredients in our food and in our water that can't be found on a label. Consumers need to take it upon themselves to check labels and to think about what possibly could be in or on the foods and products that they are putting inside their bodies. Everything you put in your body is going to have a short- or long-term impact.

I want to encourage people to take interest in their health and their child's health by being proactive, by learning, by researching, by asking more questions about specific ingredients, and by seeking help from outside sources.

A cautionary note. There are ingredients that are not listed at all but that are a concern. You might be thinking that it's overdoing it to constantly worry or think about the potential harm some of the things you ingest on a regular basis could be causing you. But, the threat is real because so many things are not regulated.

Whom can you trust?

Who may not be deserving of your trust?

It is a life process to make informed decisions about the products and foods you choose to ingest and those you choose to use on our body.

You Have Choices

The good news is there are so many choices out there. There has been a revolution in medicine of natural remedies and therapies that have come out within the past ten years and increasingly over the past five years. Many of these natural products are undergoing specific studies. I have also become aware of the growing number of websites and resources that inform about and support the use of natural remedies.

The quality of products has significantly improved over the past five years. For example, there are third-party companies testing the quality of products produced by essential oil companies. There is an essential oil company that is harvesting the essential oils only from the areas that are endemic for that specific plant, making it safe enough for you to take internally as well. That is proof to me.

At an essential oil conference, I was impressed to learn about the quality of our current essential oils. They are not growing a frankincense tree in Utah; they are going to Africa in the area where the frankincense tree is endemic and harvesting the oil there. They have set up an essential oil distillation plant to distill the oil right then and there, so it is the purest, freshest quality. The oil is brought to the United States for packaging into bottles, labeling, and to be sold.

Additionally, they are harvesting the oils and the natural plant-based products only when the particular plant is in season. There are new innovations, new research, and new information available that are easily accessible to parents.

We have learned a lot from other countries that have stopped using certain products that we are still allowing here in the United States. We know parabens are toxic ingredients in our lotions and shampoos due to research done in other countries as well as by some organizations in the United States.

We are learning from all the research that has been done and we now have U.S.-based companies making 100 percent guaranteed nontoxic products that we use every day. This is one way you can eliminate over 300 toxins from your body and your home.

I also want to make you aware of stricter regulations around animals being given hormones and toxic products to make the meat taste better or be more tender, as well as pesticides that increase fruits and vegetables harvests. Food production is improving.

Products are always being renovated and improved every year. Organic and natural labels are under stricter rules and regulations with better compliance. We have a United States-based company that for twenty-five years has been pulverizing over thirty fruits and vegetables and putting them into vegan, gluten- and soy-free capsules. They now also include vegan Omega blends. These capsules give you the seven to thirteen servings of fruits, vegetables, and omegas we so lack in our Western diet.

Confidence and Comfort That It Will Work

For the most part, natural medicines have been and continue to be much safer, and less toxic to our bodies in my experience. Because of all this new information, the products that most natural practitioners are recommending have been increasingly improving. That gives you as a parent a lot more confidence than it did thirty years ago when you would use lavender oil but you didn't know its quality. There were no regulations around how it was being harvested. It was simply poured into a bottle by the manufacturer. You could not take it internally.

Now you should have confidence, knowing it is possible to purchase products that are pure, safe, effective, and some can even be taken internally.

That gives me great comfort that products are increasingly being improved. They are safe and effective. As mentioned, there is much more research on the products and protocols.

After several thousand patients have successfully used a particular natural remedy, a protocol is established. There are clinics, for example, that are only using nutrition to treat certain types of cancers. They have a protocol in place for the plant-based remedy that they have perfected through the years and have already used successfully hundreds of times before on the particular type of cancer.

You can go with confidence to clinics in and outside of the United States where the practitioners will tell you how many people have been successfully treated with a plant-based protocol for your type of cancer over the duration that the protocol has been in place. That is important to know— helpful, and reassuring.

When I saw that, I thought to myself as a pediatrician, I don't diagnose and treat cancer in the office or in the hospital setting because I am not a pediatric cancer specialist. If there is enough information for treating a patient's cancer with a plant-based remedy, and there is, there is also enough information and research for me to treat your child's common medical ailment with a plant-based remedy and protocol.

This is what gave me the driving force to do this and to offer my services to others.

With all this past experience, there is increased confidence that these products are safe and effective because so many people have been open to the idea of using natural remedies, and they have been successful. There is a safety profile being generated on each product more than there was in the past.

THE GOD-GIVEN BLESSING OF PARENTING YOUR CHILD

Anyone who is a parent, or anyone who is close to someone who is a parent, must have felt the miracle of the gift of life. What a miracle it is as a woman to be able to give birth to a new life. For most mothers, there is an innate connection made when she looks into her baby's eyes for the first time.

To be able to continue to be a part of this other person's life, to have such influence in someone else's life is a gift from the Universe, and to know you brought forth this life into the world. That is huge for me, and that is why I want to help parents heal their children so they can have the best quality of life possible.

Parents have the power to help their child either be disease-free or to succumb to an illness that could easily be prevented by such things as lifestyle choices. A child is helpless without an adult to guide them, feed them, and love them.

To me, children are a gift from heaven. It's how heaven blesses us: the gift of procreation for ourselves and our individual lifetime, and also for humans to continue to exist into the future. I want to be able to honor that and respect that blessing by guiding parents in helping their children.

The information, the talent, and the choices I have made have brought into my life the gift of knowing pediatric health and health solutions. I want to honor parents by sharing that knowledge with them. I want to honor my Divinity by sharing the knowledge I have been blessed with so that the children of this generation and future generations are healthier.

Experiences, Ideas, and Emotions Can Contribute to Diseases

In my years of working in the office and in the hospital, there were many children I saw from birth at the hospital up to the age of eighteen. I was their sole pediatrician during the first eighteen years of their lives. It was so nice and enlightening for me to see this child growing up and learning the family dynamics.

I noticed an association in families that had a certain emotional dynamic going on, either because of a life situation happening to them or because of an emotional situation due to the child's disease.

I noticed a particular issue with children who were involved in a high-stress family situation where their parents were moving often or they were switching back and forth between parenting styles or they had to change schools multiple times. What I noticed was they had a higher probability of having an emotional disconnect from people because the people that were around them—whether it was parents, family, caretakers, or teachers in the school—were always changing.

Different environmental experiences bring up a multitude of potential emotions in each person. Our mindset connection to our emotions can contribute to stress in our lives. Stress is the beginning of so many diseases.

As I listed in Chapter Two, there are certain emotions that lead to specific diseases in our bodies. You can refer back to that chapter to have a greater understanding how childhood emotions and their environment are going to create diseases; a child's emotions and external experiences are also going to create the type of human being he or she will be, the personality he or she will have as an adult. It is all based on experiences and emotions.

As a parent, I think we have an increasing responsibility and blessing to help our children be the best adults they can be by helping influence and navigate the emotional experiences and environmental changes that they go through when they are growing up under our care.

Fulfillment of Your Legacy as a Parent

If you believe that your parenthood has been a blessing from Divinity, you want to help your child as much as possible be the healthiest, happiest, safest individual that they can be. The best, safest, and most effective way I know to do that can be accomplished by using plant-based natural remedies. Helping them find natural, non-toxic solutions to their diseases or ailments is a way of giving back to Divinity as a thank you and fulfillment of your legacy as a parent.

GETTING SUPPORT

Become Informed by Reading and Researching

One of the ways I have discovered to give thanks to Divinity for the blessing of being a parent is by informing myself of all the natural plant-based remedies I can use for the majority of common childhood diseases. I want to encourage you to do the same with your child.

I am here as a resource for you to do just that. You can go about it by researching and going to seminars and conferences on your own, like I did. You can purchase books, and talk to doctors, physicians, and nurses that have experience with this. If you have the time, desire, and trust in yourself to do that, there is plenty of information available to do it on your own. It is time consuming, but if you have the desire and confidence and you understand the information, you can do it on your own.

Lots of people have healed themselves, and I have learned that people create their own protocols for a specific ailment they had because they liked doing it all on their own.

Working One-On-One with Me and Doing My Program

You are free to do this on your own. It is time consuming and may or may not be the most cost-effective way for you to approach natural remedies because you will be dealing with a lot of trial and error on your own.

The time consumption could mean time wasted when your child gets sick. You would have to miss work getting him or her to doctors' appointments, and by doing the research yourself at home, or by attending conferences. Additionally, your child would miss days of school since he or she would likely have to be at home for a few days until the right therapy or remedy is found.

To avoid all of that, I have created a program in which I consult with parents. You would have an initial forty-five-minute consultation where we would map out the plan for your child's care. Then we would decide approximately how long that would take. It might mean anywhere from one time to several times over several weeks.

On average, I find most people, if they want to resolve a health issue permanently, need about four to twelve weeks using my mind, body, spirit practices to create simple lifestyle changes. This can take at least a month, but usually takes as long as twelve weeks, or more if it is a chronic problem. I would guide you step by step. It would be individualized, just for your child and your family's health and wellness needs.

My recommendation is the mind, body, spirit practices and lifestyle changes because it isn't just taking care of a specific disease or ailment that your child is suffering. Part of a good health program for your child is working with someone who is proactively involved in your child's health. This includes anticipatory guidance about what to do should the next problem occur so you would know ahead of time what to use if a cut becomes infected, for example.

That way, the lifestyle changes help you in the future. Not only are you decreasing your chances of letting the cut become infected, but also in case it does happen, you have already learned what to do for it ahead of time. There are only about five to ten natural plant-based products that a person can have in their cupboards to use for the majority of health issues. That has been super wonderful for me to know.

I have created a travel bag of ten products for every time I go out of town domestically or internationally. I bring this travel bag with me so I am prepared for almost any ailment that can happen while away from home. I don't have to rush to a pharmacy to purchase anything that has potentially harmful ingredients. That has been a great blessing. I don't think I could have done that with traditional Western medicine.

Thank You for Being Open to the Ideas in This Book

I know that the ideas in this book may challenge a lot of you who are used to the traditional ideas of medicine and healing that you experienced growing up in the system. Not everyone likes change, but by opening your heart to the possibilities, you will find that there are many non-toxic solutions and many more safe and effective treatments than you could ever imagine.

I want to thank you also because some of you might not have ever heard of this before. It's even more difficult to conceptualize because it takes time to get used to a new idea. I hope to honor you by offering my assistance as much as I can to help move you further toward health, whether you have heard of natural remedies before or not.

Conclusion

You are right to be concerned about toxic ingredients and negative side effects. I hope that the knowledge of the variety of natural remedies and therapies available to you has provided the guidance you need to move toward optimum health for your family and yourself.

As mentioned, natural therapies include protocols beyond products; there are many modalities beyond what I have listed in the book.

My final advice or wisdom for you is to seek help, to ask more questions, to be proactively involved, to learn as much as you can, whether you do it on your own through research or by seeking other professionals to help you.

There are many practitioners in many realms that can help you with your child's health. I would be honored if you chose to work with me.

Last, but not least: please know that you are not alone. The answer is out there, and someone else has experienced the same thing. Pray, affirm, and reach out to me! It would be my honor to help you or another healthcare practitioner who is familiar with your situation. Help is here!

The doctor of the future will give no medicine,
but will interest his or her patients
in the care of the human frame, in a proper diet,
and in the cause and prevention of disease.
~ Thomas Edison

Next Steps

It's not easy to get beyond the frustration of the trial and error of traditional Western medicine remedies that keep you stuck. If you want to transition to a healthier lifestyle and to all natural therapies, the first steps are often the most difficult, but you don't have to go it alone.

Whether you choose one-on-one consultations, telemedicine appointments, a home visit, or my twelve-week child wellness consultation program; all are designed specifically for a strong start by defining your child's health, your family's health goals, and moving you forward toward that goal.

I'd like to invite you to visit my website, naturalsolutionswithdrruth.com, or email me for more information at info@naturalsolutionswithdrruth.com.

If you are ready to schedule your one-on-one consultation call, you can do so directly with me at scheduleonce.com/meetDrRuth. If you are local to the central or south Florida area, you can meet me for half- or full-day, in-person intensives where I would consult and advise you on how to improve your child's health and make a plan for you and your family's future health with all natural remedies, including an in-home "Medicine Cabinet Makeover" and iTovi scan for yourself or a child.

You can also like my Facebook page to stay connected and receive information regarding upcoming events and classes. Additionally, I share information on children's health and wellness issues at facebook.com/page/ naturalsolutionswithDrRuth. I also regularly write articles for *Natural Awakenings* magazine, Space & Treasure Coast edition: naturalawakeningsmag.com, and teach monthly group classes in different locations throughout the fifty states.

Let me help guide you on your search for your children's wellness with all natural solutions. Thank you for being a part of this journey with me.

About the Author

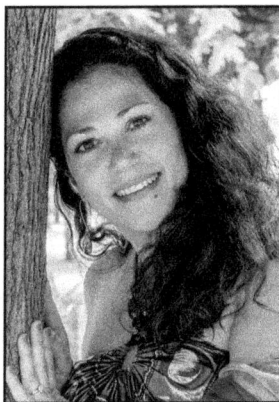

Dr. Ruth Rodriguez is a Board Certified Osteopathic Pediatrician, wife, mother of two, a half-marathon runner, and a soon to be published author. She has a passion for using natural solutions to improve the overall health of the families she sees, as well as providing the necessary information for their holistic wellness needs.

With her personal and professional experience of over twenty-three years of clinical work in both inpatient and outpatient pediatric healthcare, she has developed a twelve-week, step-by-step program of exercise, diet, and natural supplements.

Dr. Ruth's work has not only helped herself and her family. She has empowered others to take control of their own and their children's health through her recommendations of plant-based therapies, including transitioning from medications to all-natural supplements, body, home, and healthcare products.

In addition, she helps her patients holistically by guiding them in the use of spiritual and mindfulness practices, counseling, and other alternative medicine pediatric advice.

Notes

Notes